LOOKING GOOD AND FEELING GOOD

Weight Loss Guide to Better Health and Wellness

Kay Whiting

BookLeaf Publishing Company, LLC.

4321 Kingwood Drive, Suite 104

Kingwood, Texas 77365

ISBN 978-1-941031-30-8

First Printing, 2014

Printed in the United States of America

No claims are made as to how much weight you can lose using this information/product. Your results will vary from any examples given. Your total weight loss will depend upon your circumstances, the amount of calories that you consume on a daily basis, your determination, your activity level, and the duration of your efforts to lose weight.

Liability Disclaimer

By reading this document, you assume all risks associated with using the advice given below, with a full understanding that you, solely, are responsible for anything that may occur as a result of putting this information into action in any way, and regardless of your interpretation of the advice.

You further agree that our company cannot be held responsible in any way for the success or failure of your business as a result of the information presented below. It is your responsibility to conduct your own due diligence regarding the safe and successful operation of your business if you intend to apply any of our information in any way to your business operations.

Terms of Use

You are given a non-transferable, "personal use" license to this product. You cannot distribute it or share it with other individuals.

Also, there are no resale rights or private label rights granted when purchasing this document. In other words, it's for your own personal use only.

LOOKING GOOD AND FEELING GOOD

Weight Loss Guide to Better Health and Wellness

Kay Whiting

"The higher your energy level, the more efficient your body. The more efficient your body, the better you feel and the more you will use your talent to produce outstanding results. "

- Anthony Robbins

Thank You!
I wanted to just take the time to **"Thank You"** personally for investing in yourself and I really hope you will follow the steps in this book to achieve your goals.

Can You Help Me Out?
When you get a free second, could you be kind enough to leave an honest review on Amazon.com about this book. I am always looking for feedback so I can improve my content to better help you. Thank you in advance for your help.

Table of Contents

Weight Loss The Healthy Way

When you are beginning a diet program you are probably wondering how you will able to do it in a healthy manner. Well you need to begin your journey to weight loss, by assessing your own needs, because no two diet programs will work the same for everyone. You should begin by taking stock of your emotional and physical conditions which can possibly interfere with your weight loss goals. It is a good practice to visit your doctor before you even consider your weight loss program. He will be able to tell you if you are healthy enough to undergo the weight loss in general.

You will also find that a lot of the weight loss experts suggest that you create a healthy diet plan along with plenty of physical activity for you to have a healthy weight loss. You need to make sure you have plenty of vitamins, minerals, and proteins. You should also plan on lower calories, but not in essential elements for remaining healthy.

You should also be aware that your body will require a certain amount of these vitamins and minerals for it to remain healthy as well as

3

function well. A healthy diet will supply your body with all of the vitamins and minerals that it will need. Both problems and disorders will definitely arise, if you do not supply your body with the essential elements. By maintaing these healthy amounts you will lose one to two pounds a week, but no more.

Another thing that will affect your healthy weight loss is the lack of sleep. When you do not get the right amount of sleep it will slow down your metabolism which will make it harder to lose or maintain your weight. Lack of sleep will also raise your Cortisol levels which will result in increased appetite and increased cravings for sugar which will lead to weight gain.

The Glycemic index is the measurement of impact that carbohydrates have on sugar. The carbohydrates that will break down sugar slowly in your body will encourage stable blood sugars which will allow them to rate low on the Glycemic index. For you to have a healthy weight loss you need to become familiar with the glycemic value of the certain foods that you eat as well as staying away from the bad carb foods. If your diet includes more good carbs it will help you keep your appetite in check and help you maintain healthy sugar levels.

All of these are some of the most important steps that you will need to take in order to maintain healthy weight loss methods. The more you work towards a healthy weight loss, the healthier you will be and the more energy you will have.

Weight Gain Can Ensure Health and Fitness

People—especially those who are very thin for their frame, age, and height—would be very happy upon discovering that they have gained some weight. For them, this weight gain would indicate not only the condition of their health and fitness but also the improvements on their physical built as well.

Aside from being an indicator of good health, fitness, and eating a well-balanced diet, weight gain would also serves an indicator for a person's overall improvement in his or her outlook in life. Although in most cases, weight gain is an indicator of good health, it can also serve as an indicator if negligence especially if there are signs of obesity.

To know if weight gain is bad or good for you, it is always best to conduct a research about its indicators as well as of its advantages and disadvantages so you will have an idea if you're into the right thing.

What you need to know?

Weight gain refers to the increase in a person's body weight brought by intake of too many calories, lack of physical activity such as regular exercise, or a side effect of certain types of medication. However, it can also be a result of a certain set of workout routine—such as those in bodybuilding—wherein muscles tend to increase in terms of weight.

Experts say that weight gain is usually done by people because of two reasons. One, they want to build muscles for a fit body. This is very common to people who need big muscles for their jobs such gym instructors, fitness gurus, bodybuilding coaches, bouncers, bodyguards, weightlifters, and the like.

The second reason why people gain weight is because of their health. Weight gain is highly recommended to those people who have lost so much body fat due to dieting and especially to those who have developed various eating disorders such as anorexia or bulimia. People—especially women who are believed to suffer more from this condition—are advised to gain weight to recover from all the body fats and nutrients they have lost.

To know if you are gaining some weight, check for its symptoms such as a rounder belly, certain increase in the fat percentage of the body, increased mass of muscles and increase in the level of body's hydration. Experts say that it can be hard to determine if a person's weight gain is good or not. This is because people have different individual needs that need to be paid attention to. Although knowing the ideal weight for a person's height can be a god indicator, it is always best to consult with a physician to avoid further complications. For those who are planning to gain weight to ensure them health and fitness, here are some helpful tips to get by:

1. Set your focus on set of workouts routines that target how one can increase body fat and muscles. This is one of the most effective ways of gaining weight without having to worry about obesity. Since a person burns only the unnecessary fats, he or she is paving the way for the muscles to gain weight.

2. Spend some time for to know what the target weight gain is. Just like in losing weight, weight gain also requires utmost time and dedication. If one is into weight gain, he or she must make sure that they are serious about it so they will get their desired health and level of fitness.

3. Always have a healthy and well balanced diet. For people who are gaining weight for health and fitness, this is very important if because it serves as their guide on what kind of food they should eat and the proper amount of each to get the weight that they desire.

Weight Loss Advice

If you are like many you are trying hard to lose weight. You have tried almost every diet pill and program that is available to no avail. The harder you seemed to try the more you seemed to fail.

You are ready to give up and don't know where else to turn. You feel lost and alone. You may even feel ashamed because you failed at your weight loss. Well there is no reason that you need to feel this way as there are some tips that you can follow to achieve your weight loss goals.

1. Exercise:
In order for you to be successful in your weight loss you need to do plenty of exercise. You should work out at least 30 minutes a day to achieve the best results. Your exercise does not have to be a grueling unfriendly task. It can be something you enjoy such as taking a walk with a friend, swimming, or even playing tennis are some great ways for you to get your exercise that you need. The more you exercise the more calories that you will burn. It is also great for your overall general health.

2. Diary:

A diary will help you stay on schedule with your weight loss goals. It can also reveal some very amazing information on your weight loss goals such as how much weight you have already lost. It may even be able to tell your trigger points that cause you to binge. All of these will help you be aware and get closer to your weight loss goals.

3. Lose weight slowly:
Most weight loss experts recommend that you do not lose more than one or two pounds a week depending on your overall body size. The more quickly you lose your weight. The more likely that it will return.

4. Balanced diet:
A balanced diet is important to any weight loss goals. A diet that is rich in fruits, vegetables, grains, and lean meats are all great to reach your weight loss goals. Also eating 6 small meals compared to 3 big ones will help you fight the in between meal cravings.

5. Skipping meals:
It is important that you are not skipping meals especially breakfast. Breakfast is one of the most important meals of the day as it jump starts your metabolism. Also avoiding skipping meals will help your body avoid those nasty cravings.

These are just some of the tips that you can follow for a healthy weight loss.

14

Weight Loss Calorie Counter

Do you want to find a good weight loss calorie counter? You want a program or book that lists both the calorie content of foods eaten and of ways you burn the energy off. That's why it's important to find a dual featured weight loss calorie counter.

If you are trying to lose weight, you probably aren't very good at judging the impact of food and exercise on your body's shape. Whether you are a beginning dieter or have struggled with your weight for some time, you have to develop an idea of how many calories are in food and how many calories you are burning.

Take this quick quiz: which has the fewest calories: A fast food meal or a meal ordered at a restaurant? With all of the bashing burger chains get, you'd never know that most people actually eat fewer calories at these places than they would at a sit down restaurant. That's why it doesn't do to go by "common sense." You need a reliable weight loss calorie counter.

Everyone knows that in order to lose weight, you have to burn more calories than you consume. But too many people believe they eat fewer calories than they actually consume and they also overestimate how many calories they burn in any given situation. That is why having a weight loss calorie counter is so important.

Here are some features of a good weight loss calorie counter.

Your weight loss calorie counter needs to include a wide range of foods. These should include whole foods such as apples, potatoes, and 3 ounces of lean beef. But, it should also include common recipes and combinations of foods. Further, it should include processed food such as chips and packaged cookies. Ideally, your weight loss calorie counter will include common fast food and restaurant items as well.

Just like your nutrition weight loss calorie counter needs to have a wide variety of foods listed, your exercise software should include a wide array of activities. Many such programs include a wide range of what we would consider "exercise" such as high impact aerobics, lifting weights, and swimming as well as leisure activities that involve physical activity including bicycling, table tennis, and recreational volleyball. Some go even further and list things like playing with kids, standing, reading, etc.

When it comes to calories burned, it's not as simple as saying "running a mile burns 98 calories." That statement happens to be true if you are 150 pounds. But, a 120 pound woman will only burn 78 calories in that distance and a 180 pound man will burn 117 calories. That's because the body mass has an impact on calories burned. So, when looking for a weight loss calorie counter, find one that takes your weight into consideration.

First you need to acknowledge the need for a book or computer program that tells you exactly how many calories are involved with any activity. Then you need one that covers the wide range of foods and activities you do. Finally, you need to find one that takes your weight into account. That's how you find a weight loss calorie counter.

Weight Loss For The Obese

If you are trying for weight loss pounds, you are not alone. Some people need to lose a few pounds. But more and more Americans are in the categories known as obese and morbidly obese. These people need to lose more than a few lbs. They need weight loss pounds.

Some people have been able to have a significant weight loss pounds through diet and exercise. This is made popular by television shows such as The Biggest Loser.

These kinds of people are able to change their attitude and lifestyle for life. They realize that they're not on a temporary diet. To weight loss pounds, they must change how they view their body and the food they eat.

This means they change the types and quantity of food they buy. They change the types of meals they eat. They change the size of the meals they eat. They change the frequency of the meals they eat.

And, they begin to exercise. Because they may be unable to do vigorous activity, they may have to start slowly. But, morbidly obese people should choose to exercise at least 30 minutes a day in whatever form is possible. As they develop strength and endurance, they should kick this up to 60 to 90 minutes.

But some people feel they cannot change their habits on their own. The weight loss pounds are not realistic with just diet and exercise. That is why Bariatric Surgery has become so popular in the last few years.

With this procedure, also known as Gastric Bypass, the stomach is made significantly smaller and the food bypasses part of the small intestine. People who have undergone this surgery find that they feel full with very small portions of food.

In a Roux-en-Y gastric bypass (the most common kind); the stomach is made smaller by creating a small pouch at the top of the stomach using surgical staples or a plastic band. The smaller stomach is connected directly to the middle portion of the small intestine bypassing the rest of the stomach and the upper portion of the small intestine.

Gastric bypass surgeries may cause what is known as the "dumping syndrome." This happens when food moves too rapidly through the stomach and intestines. Symptoms include nausea, weakness, sweating, faintness, and sometimes diarrhea shortly after eating. These symptoms are much more severe when the person has eaten highly refined, high-calorie foods, especially sweets.

There are a number of weight loss pounds conditions that have to be met before a doctor can perform Gastric bypass. For instance, the person has to have been obese for at least 5 years. He or she cannot have an ongoing problem with alcohol or have untreated depression. Most candidates are between 18 and 65 years old.

Most people who have gastric bypass surgery quickly begin to lose weight. They tend to continue to lose weight for up to 12 months. One study showed that most patients will lose about one-third of their original body weight in 1 to 4 years. However, if the recommended diet is not followed properly, the patient can begin to stretch their stomach and weight may be regained.

Strict lifestyle changes and gastric bypass surgery are two options for quick weight loss pounds.

Weight Loss After Pregnancy

When you are pregnant you normally will gain on average approximately 25 to 30 pounds. When the baby is born, however you may find yourself needing to lose about 25 to 30 pounds of excess weight shortly after giving birth. If you eat as close to natural as much as you possibly can is one of the best ways that you can lose weight after your pregnancy and be able to keep it off. To put it simply you will see better results for a longer period of time when you are steering clear of the processed foods and focus on making wise and healthy food choices.

1. Fruits:
Any type of fruit whether its natural or canned are great for helping you shed extra weight. The fruits are low in sodium and therefore they are also good for reducing your risks of heart disease as well as high blood pressure. The canned or frozen fruit are a great choice because you will not have to eat them right away as you would with the fresh fruit. They are just as nutritious and good for you.

2. Vegetables:

Vegetables will also help reduce the chances of high cholesterol and blood pressure. They also help destroy cancer causing radicals and are full of fiber. They can be eaten fresh, canned or frozen because they are packaged to seal in the much needed vitamins and minerals. You can lose some of the vital nutrients however so you will need to be careful how you cook them.

3. Breastfeeding:

Breastfeeding may actually aid in your weight loss. This is because breastfeeding releases certain hormones into your body that will help your uterus contract and return to its pre-pregnancy size and shape faster than a woman who does not breastfeed. Sometimes however, you will not lose the excess weight till after you have stopped breast feeding because you will need to take in extra calories.

4. Water:

This is an important part for losing weight because it will increase your metabolism and help stop your food cravings. If you are already eating plenty of fruits and vegetables you are also consuming a lot of water as well. It is still good for you to drink 6-8 glasses of water a day though.

5. Exercise:

This will help aid in your postpartum weight loss and help you to minimize your postpartum depression. Along with the exercise you should also eat a healthy diet that is low in fat but full of vitamins and minerals and also is high in fiber. You should exercise 30 minutes a day five days a week to see an appropriate weight loss.

These are all great tips for you to use when you are trying to lose your pregnancy weight. You need to be sure to begin in moderation though so that your body can acclimate to the change in your routine.

Weight Loss Drugs

Most available weight loss drugs in the market today need doctor's prescription. There are weight loss drugs that are bought over the counter without doctor's prescription but the general rule is to always consult with the doctors first before taking in any medication for weight loss.

Natural weight loss programs are always more advisable than weight loss drugs. Healthier diet, regular exercise, and a change in the ways of living are always better than resorting to medicines or weight loss drugs.

Although many weight loss drugs can help in reducing weight, proper care must be taken to ensure the effectiveness. There are studies that show that weight loss drugs may be harmful to health in the long run and may cause side effects like diarrhea, headaches, dizziness, and increase blood pressure.

The two most commonly available weight loss drugs today are Orlistat and Sibrutamine. The prices of these drugs vary from $130-$200 for a month dosage. They have been reported to cause side effects and are mostly prescribed to people who need to lose weight for health or medical related reasons.

Orlistat is an inhibitor of fat absorption in the body. The most prestigious brand for Orlistat is Xenical. This is a worldwide popular weight loss drug that has received several testimonials from users. Most users complain of oil in their bowels, stomach ache and uncontrollable bowel movement. Despite this, Orlistat has been known to be a very effective weight loss drug as it instills discipline among users. People using Orlistat will be forced to visit the toilet more if they eat fatty food. Therefore, the less fat they take in, the more controlled and easy their bowel movements are going to be. In the long run, when the body is used to denying fatty food, the better weight maintenance could be attained.

Weight loss drugs can certainly fast track weight loss but it is important to note that it should always be accompanied by proper diet and a regular exercise. Weight loss drugs taken without correct low calorie and low cholesterol diet may cause complications without proper care and medical consultation.

The value of reducing food intake cannot be overstressed. Drinking water is the best way to trick hunger pangs. Water is a natural food suppressant. There are also some medicines that are appetite suppressants. Redux is one of the most popular weight loss drugs that suppress appetite. This drug is made of phentermine combined with fenfluramine. Fenfluramine was taken out from the market back in the 90's because it has been proven to cause damages to heart valves. Phentermine, however, is still available but can only be bought under strict medical prescription.

Taking drugs for weight loss is not a bad thing. For some people, it is highly recommended specially if the need to lose weight is dire and the time needed for the weight loss is immediate. For people who only want to lose weight for cosmetics reason, a natural weight loss plan which includes low-calorie diet, increase water intake, and regular exercises is still safer with long term effects.

Weight Loss Pills

Weight loss pills are the fad today. People worldwide are trying to find ways to quickly lose weight. In the US alone, 70 million men and women search for diet pills and other easy and affordable weight reduction drugs.

Several studies have been made to test different weight loss pills available in the market. Some studies show that two of the most effective herbal weight loss pills are those that contain green tea extracts and bitter orange. Green tea is popular for the natural antioxidants found in them. Antioxidants get rid of toxins and burn calories and fats. Bitter oranges are citrus fruits that have been used by traditional Chinese herbalists for medical purposes. This fruit contains different chemicals including synephrine which is said to be effective chemical that can promote weight loss.

There are hundreds of weight loss pills being sold to public without government health clearances. This poses great danger to health and may even result in mortality. Wight loss pills effectiveness may be popular. However, everyone should also be aware that taking supplementary diet pills are risky and may even be fatal.

Health experts still strongly recommend natural weight loss programs instead of speeding up weight loss by using weight loss pills. According to a consultation with a doctor, the herbal weight loss pills available in the market today may cause severe damage to kidneys because the dosage on the pill may not be controlled or regulated.

Several occasions of lung and kidney failures have been reported as side effects of weight loss pills. There have been reported cases of heart attacks, strokes and even death. Unknown to many people, some natural ingredients found in herbal weight loss pills contain chemicals that might cause death.

There was a time when herbal diet pills became popular in the US. People were looking for a supplementary food that will increase energy and help them lose weight. Ephedra became famous for this. Ephedra or otherwise called Sea Grape or Ma Huang, is a shrub that is a main ingredient of most weight loss pills during 1990s. Since it was sold and marketed as a natural supplementary diet pill, people thought it was safe.

Several years after Ephedra came out in the market, the Federal Drug Agency (FDA) received reports Ephedra can cause heart attacks and death. Since FDA had limited powers, the only thing the agency was able to do is to recommend a sign on the packages stating that the product should be discontinued after 7 days of use.

In 2003, an American athlete died after working out. Steve Bechler was a pitcher for Baltimore Orioles. Steve was using pills that contained Ephreda. Soon after that, US government banned the sale of weight loss pills that contained Ephedra.

This is just one of the many reported issues related to weight loss pills. There are different ways to lose weight. Weight loss pills are no substitute to a healthier diet, regular exercise and enough sleep. Do not take the easy way of losing weight and get in trouble. Lose weight the healthier way and enjoy life.

Weight Loss Pills and Their Effects

There are many lose weight pills on the market. They tout numerous benefits and list a variety of substances. But the layperson doesn't really know what kinds of effects these supplements have in them. Therefore, I turned to the highly respected Mayo Medical Clinic to find out what the effectiveness of the items in the lose weight pills were.

The hot trend in lose weight pills is Bitter Orange. This is touted in many supplements as an "ephedra substitute. There is some scientific thinking that it may cause similar problems as ephedra – which was pulled off the market for causing heart attack and stroke. There hasn't been enough research on Bitter Orange and the long term effects are unknown.

Chitosan is described as a relatively safe ingredient in supplements. The manufacturers often tout this as having the ability to block the absorption of fat into the body. Mayo says this is highly unlikely. Also, they caution that it may cause constipation and bloating. Again, the long term effects are unknown.

Chromium is another of the lose weight pills that is relatively safe but unlikely to work according to Mayo. It supposedly reduces body fat and builds muscle.

CLA can cause diarrhea and indigestion. Mayo says it might be able to decrease fat and increase muscle, but is unlikely to reduce overall body weight.

Country Mallow is supposed to decrease appetite and increase the number of calories burned. But, like Bitter Orange, it contains ephedra and has all of the associated risks.

Ephedra has been banned for medical or supplement use, but is still allowed to be sold as a tea. Despite this, many supplements still contain ephedra. It can cause high blood pressure, heart rate irregularities, sleeplessness, seizures, heart attacks, strokes and even death and should be strenuously avoided.

Green tea extract is included in any number of lose weight pills. It is supposed to increase calorie burning and metabolism and decrease appetite. There is limited evidence to support this claim, according to Mayo. However, it can cause vomiting, bloating, indigestion and diarrhea. Also, it contains a high amount of caffeine, so if you are watching that, you may want to restrict supplements containing Green tea.

Guar Gum is another supplement that is harmless but unlikely to cause any real weight loss. Makers claim that it blocks the absorption of dietary fat and increases the feeling of fullness, which leads to decreased calorie intake. However, it is more likely to cause diarrhea, flatulence and other gastrointestinal problems.

Finally, Hoodia is another ingredient found in many weight loss pills. It is supposed to decrease appetite. However, the Mayo Clinic says there is no conclusive evidence to support this claim.

Many people have found success using these types of supplements. However, they are expensive and there are no legitimate scientific studies that back up the claims. These lose weight pills are quite expensive, so you have to balance the payoff versus the payout.

Weight Loss For Teenage Girls

Weight loss for teenage girls is a hot topic these days as so many teenagers are trying to look like their celebrity idols. What they fail to realize is that most pictures of celebrities have been airbrushed to make the woman look thinner and more beautiful. Add to that the bevy of hairstylists and other professionals on hand prior to the photo shoot and it is easy to see why girls are so misled. It is a pity that they couldn't see their favorite celebrity in all her morning glory i.e. without makeup or hairstylists as then they would get a truer picture.

So what type of weight loss for teenage girls is healthy? Some teenage girls need to lose weight and get more exercise. In fact about a fifth of the teenage population is severely overweight and that carries long term health risks. They are more likely to suffer cardiac problems, diabetes and a whole host of other illnesses.

Other teenagers are underweight with anorexia and bulimia being an issue amongst girls and boys. Regardless of your child's weight issues, never let their weight become a focus point. Life is too short to obsess over weight gain or loss unless it is causing a potentially serious health problem. Then you need advice from a suitably qualified doctor, not your friends and neighbors; regardless of how well meaning they may be.

All teenagers would benefit from a healthy lifestyle program. They need to eat better and exercise more. Don't forget that kids learn from their parents so if you are not fit, active and eating healthily then you can't expect your kids to be. The whole family should change their diet at the same time as this is less likely to cause teenagers to become obsessive over their weight.

Educate your kids about the different food groups. Explain the different roles that carbohydrates, protein and fats make up in their body. Don't prohibit any particular food as that will immediately make it more attractive. But that doesn't mean that they can have candy and cakes every day. Suggest that these remain a treat for special occasions.

Take your teenager shopping with you and allow them to pick out their meals based on some light ground rules such as lean meat and must include at least two fruit or vegetables. Teach them how to cook their own food so that they do not rely on pre-packaged or worse fast food pickups.

Get your teenagers involved in sports. Hopefully they will have played some form since childhood but if they haven't yet found something they enjoy, encourage them to sign up for some classes. You may have to "bribe" them with the lure of a new outfit or night out at bowling or the movies (skipping the soda pop and candy obviously!).

Exercise is great for all of us and helps with weight loss for teenage girls. It also helps them to deal with their hormones and other aspects of growing up.

Weight Loss For All Teens

In today's society, which is full of peer pressure, there are many teens that are feeling peer pressure to lose weight. You need to be aware, though that if you happen to be one of these teenagers, that you need to be sure you are losing the weight for the right reasons.

Which include for you to be happy and healthy, not just in an effort for you to be popular? If you happen to be a teen that is overweight and you are trying to lose weight, it is best for you if you lose the weight slowly and naturally.

Here are some real easy tips for you that might help you achieve your weight loss goals. These tips will also help you lose weight slowly as well as naturally.

1. Eating slower:
When you eat slower you are increasing your chances of losing weight. A lot of people especially teenagers tend to forget to chew their food completely before swallowing and it enters their stomach too quickly. You need to remember that food needs to be broken down into tiny

43

pieces in order for you to get all the nutrients. Be sure you take the time and chew your food thoroughly. Chewing your food completely will help you burn calories faster as well.

2. Junk food:
Another great tip for you is for you to ditch the junk food. Junk food is jam packed with tons of sodium, sugars, and calories which will add to your waistline and also your blood pressure and cholesterol levels. Try replacing these foods with such things with natural fruits and vegetables. You can even do searches online for a list of foods that will aid in burning fat faster.

3. Water:
It is very important that you drink plenty of water so that you can boost up your metabolism. Water will not only help you lose weight but it is also great for your pores; thanks to the minerals that it contains. The more water that you consume the happier and healthier you will be.

You need to remember though that when you begin to drink water in an effort to lose weight you need to cut out all those junk drinks. This includes soda, frapachinos and anything else that is loaded with sugars and calories. Just think you will even save money by cutting these expensive little things out of your diet. You are allowed to have a little caffeine as it helps boost the metabolism a little which will aide in your weight loss.

4. Set Monthly goals:
It is good for you to also set small monthly goals and then be sure you reach them. If you are overweight it is best for you to lose one or two pounds a week. This will help you ensure that you are well on your way to your weight loss goals in a healthy and safe manner.

These are all great tips for you to achieve your weight loss goals. You need to be careful when you are doing these to help prevent too much weight loss which can lead to serious health issues.

46

Weight Loss Plans For Teens

If you're a teenager looking for weight loss plans for teens, then you're no doubt in a very difficult moment of your life. The trick for success in losing weight is to understand and accept that whatever plan you decide is for you, and then your success will not happen overnight. So it's important to be realistic and not set yourself up for a frustrating fall.

Your first step before you jump on any weight loss plans for teens is to make sure that you have the basics down and you've tried them to the best of your abilities. That means taking regular and adequate exercise for your ability and fitness levels – increasing in frequency and level as your fitness improves. It also means cutting out fast foods and junk foods and eating a diet heavy in fresh fruits and vegetables and fiber. Also, make sure that any between meal snacking is avoided, because this is a surefire way to pile on the pounds and ruin all your good work. Drinking at least a liter and a half of water per day is also the basics of weight loss and should be actively encouraged. If you have tried these basics and you're still struggling to lose weight, then one of

47

the weight loss plans for teens might just be for you.

Whichever plan you opt for there are certain points that you should make sure the plan either includes or doesn't include. Often people say avoid fad diets because any weight loss that is achieved will reappear once the user goes back to their everyday eating plans. As much as this is true, often time's people cannot agree on what is considered a fad diet. So you will no doubt get contradictions about which group a particularly popular diet falls into.

Pretty much though, it is a matter of using your common sense and judging for yourself whether a diet program is for you. For instance judge the kind of foods that a program is asking you to eat, if those foods are overly restrictive, then you might want to look further at the program and see if it is for you.

Some weight loss plans never include the taking of regular exercise, which for anyone, whether they are looking to lose weight or not, is important. For a growing teen regular exercise is crucial, so if there is no reference to taking exercise, again ask yourself if this program would really suit you and your needs.

Weight loss plans for teens are always a good idea because finding a successful program will not only help to lose the weight, but it will also foster confidence and a high self-esteem in a growing and maturing teen.

Weight Loss For Vegetarians

Are you one of the many that have a weight problem? Are you one of the many who is dealing with obesity with the related issues that are related with being overweight such as the risk of colon problems and heart disease? Well do not feel alone there are over 60% of Americans are either overweight or obese.

A balanced diet tends to leans towards the vegetarian lifestyle. This type of diet can aide you in regulating your digestion as well as maintaining healthy cholesterol and blood sugar levels. You need to be aware though that being a vegetarian is not a short term diet it's a complete lifestyle change. The good thing is that there is research that proves a relationship between vegetarian life style, more physical activity, decreased smoking and drinking; are related to a healthier life style. Being a vegetarian also lowers the death rates from chronic disorders.

There several different types of vegetarians and you need to be aware of them.

1. Vegans and Strict Vegans-These are the ones that do not eat or use any animal products. They also avoid all fur and leather along with edible products of animal origin such as honey. Their staple diet includes such things as vegetables, fruits, legumes, grains, and seeds among others.

2. Raw Vegans-These are the vegetarians who rely largely on the raw vegan foods. These include such foods as sprouted grains and fermented foods among others. Just recently this type of diet has become popular among people because it provides a simple yet tasty weight to obtain weight loss. These types of foods also are high in fiber so people on this diet do not have attacks of hunger.

3. Lacto-ova vegetarians-This will include your dairy products and eggs in your diet as well as the fruit and vegetables. This is a great way for you to transition from being a non-vegetarian to a vegetarian diet because it is not as strict as most vegan diets.

4. Pesco-and Pollo-Vegetarians-The Pesco vegetarians will include fish into their diets whereas the pollo portion also includes chicken. Therefore these two categories cannot be considered strict vegetarians but they are strict advocates of healthy and organic food choices for a form of detoxification and also health reasons.

Regardless of the form of a vegetarian diet it gives weight loss benefits due to the calorie density that is involved. Therefore a diet that is rich in fiber will fill you up quicker and helps you curb your appetite.

You need to be aware though that even vegetarians need to keep an eye on their overall calorie intake in order to remain healthy. But it is still one of the best ways for anyone to lose weight if it is used in the correct form.

54

Weight Loss Tips That Work

There is no easy way out of obesity but there is certainly a way to beat it. As a matter of fact, you only need to remember two words if you want to lose weight: Hard Work. Face the fact, there is no substitute for hard work if you want to be successful in many aspects of life; losing weight is no exemption. It takes a lot of time, commitment, and dedication to trim down, slim down, and be healthier. With a little planning and a lot of will power, plus weight loss tips from experts, you can be on your way to a healthier you.

Whether you wish to shed just a few pounds or lose from 20 to 30 pounds, weight loss tips can make dieting, exercise, and the whole weight loss venture easier and safer for you. But remember that weight loss tips is not meant to be the only tool you can use, your effort is actually the key factor to a fast track weight loss. That being said, here are a few tips you can commit to:

Proper Diet

In contrast to popular belief, diet is not mainly concentrated on losing weight instead it is also essential for maintaining an overall healthy you.

Diet is usually defined as eating a controlled amount of certain food to regulate weight. Some people are on a diet to lose weight while many go on a diet to gain weight usually in the form of muscles. Proper diet starts with getting rid of foods which are not beneficial to the body. Cut back on fats, alcohol, and the intake of abusive drugs. Next, consult your doctor to find a diet that fits your need.

Drink Water

What better way to quench thirst than drinking a glass or more of water? Forget the frizzy drinks, sweetened fruit beverages, milkshakes, and iced teas. Compared to other drinks, water has no calories and cools your body. Drink 12-16 ounces of water every meal and bring along a bottle of water when you are on the go. If you like, you can squeeze fresh lemon for a zesty taste. This may be one of the simplest weight loss tip you can commit to, drink water and flush those unwanted fats from your body.

Exercise

Here is where hard work is really demanded. Though some people live hectic lives and the even the thought of exercising makes their body ache, exercise is a great loss weight tip to both lose weight and maintain a healthy body. Those

56

who have very demanding jobs can still exercise in their own simple ways. A daily walk to the office or from the office to your home instead of driving your car is already a form of exercise. How about taking the stairs instead of the elevator? If you have time to spare, take Aerobic exercises or do other physical activities which require more body movements. The more effort you exert, the more weight you lose.

Weight loss is achievable with will power, proper diet, water intake, and exercise. Follow these simple weight loss tips and benefit from them.

58

Weight Loss Without The Cost

I am sure you have seen the many advertisements out there for one weight loss program or another and they all are promoting weight loss in a matter of weeks. These advertisements are ranging from the simple every day diet programs to surgical procedures. I am sure you are also well aware of the one thing that these all have in common, the sky high cost.

Helping people lose weight and achieve an ideal body shape is a money making business today due to the massive demand. The gyms you may join, dieticians with hefty bills, and also the food that many of the programs suggest come with a hefty price tag. Achieving a healthy weight loss is not that hard so there is no reason why you cannot achieve the same results from these diet programs on your own and save money while doing it.

1. Know the basics-

If you want to make your own diet charts, as well as your very own exercise program, it is important that you know the science to healthy weight loss. While healthy weight loss is mainly about calorie intake it also entails the distribution of those various calories throughout the day. There are also certain conditions that you may have that may be a deterrent to your weight loss goals. In this case you will need to contact your doctor before you begin. There are several resources on the internet today such as calorie counters which can be downloaded for free and used for easy reference.

2. No gain without a little pain-

Starving should not be part of your weight loss program instead, you should practice restrictive eating. The amount of the restriction will depend on the extent of the foods that are in your diet and it will be something you need to maintain the rest of your life. You will have to give up certain foods however to reach your ideal weight goals.

3. Use it or lose it-

If you are one of the many that looks at exercise as one of those unpleasant chores that you must do, you need to be able to develop a better attitude. There are certain exercises that you do every day without even knowing about them such as playing with your kids, beach workouts, and yes even sex are good forms and fun ways of burning off those excess calories. These are the activities that are not only good for toning your body but also gives you a high like no alcohol could do and as a result you are not putting any harmful toxins into your body.

These are all great ways for you to shed those excess pounds and they are a lot cheaper than some of those that are available today. If you are trying to lose weight, but are on a tight budget; give these ideas a try.

Do You Need The Gym

The good news is that you do not need the gym for weight loss workouts. Some people have a fear of the gym particularly if they are not used to the equipment. For others, they simply don't want other people looking at them when they are exercising. This was my fear until I realized that most people down the gym is too busy getting fit to pay anyone else any attention.

Exercise is a great way to become healthier. The more muscle you build the faster your metabolism becomes. But you should always seek your doctor's opinion before embarking on workouts especially if you are severally overweight.

Try and find an exercise you enjoy. You are far more likely to do it and it will be easier to add that weight loss workout to your overall lifestyle. There are countless types of fitness activities that you can try. Riding a bike is a great way to workout providing you do it regularly. And a gentle bike through the park is not sufficient. You need to be biking up and down hills to really get the benefit from this program.

Aerobics may suit some people although be warned as it can be heavy going on your joints. Be sure to attend a class held by a qualified teacher and ask to start with low impact exercises. Always choose the right gear particularly your gym shoes as you need to protect your body. It is not a great calorie burner though despite the fact that you can end up sweating a lot. You would use up more calories climbing the stairs a lot at home.

Swimming is a great exercise if you are worried about your joints or have an injury which affects your ability to work out. You won't lose a lot of calories unless you work really hard but it is great for your heart and lungs.

You could try combining swimming and aerobics i.e. aquarobics. The water adds an element of resistance. This should help you to tone up quicker but only if the instructor makes you work harder. Gentle classes are not your goal at the moment!

Pilates is a fantastic exercise for those looking for weight loss workouts. The simple mechanics of Pilates make you stand straighter; this automatically makes you look like you have lost weight. Good instructors will help you to advance to more specific Pilates moves to help you tone more quickly without causing injury.

Walking is a great way to get some free exercise. Buy a cheap pedometer to keep track of those steps. You want to aim for at least 10,000 per day. Swinging your arms as you walk will encourage you to walk faster and thus burn more calories. We are not looking at going for a gentle stroll. Leave that to the older folk. Walking helps prevent heart disease and stroke.

There are so many choices available for weight loss workouts; you will easily find one to suit your needs.

Online Weight Loss Programs

So you are looking at trying to lose weight and are unsure on what to do next. Are you going to go it alone or are you going to want to join a weight loss program. If you happen to decide on a weight loss program, you then need to choose if you wish to go to one in your own local area or find one to join online. A lot of these online programs have become real popular but each option has both its good and its bad elements. Here are a few of the elements that will hopefully help you decide which type of program is the right one for you.

When you are attending a local weight loss group or other diet center, you will have the opportunity for face to face accountability; for the weight that you either lose or do not lose. This is a good option for you if you are worried about whether or not you will cheat on your diet or even if you need someone else to push you along. It will be harder for you to cheat on your diet, when you know you will have to come face to face with someone; as well as answer for your own actions.

Another great advantage to the local diet centers is it will give you the opportunity to meet new people and be able to discuss either your success or your failures with them. When you are dieting it is much easier to go through it with other people who are going through the same thing.

The one drawback, of the local diet centers, is the face to face interaction; which may keep you from attending these centers. You also may be too embarrassed to join one of these programs because of your overall weight.

If you are one that does happen to be embarrassed or even uncomfortable with the idea of meeting other people, then the online option will probably be better for you. Just for the fact that the internet provides you the total privacy that you may desire.

Another great advantage is that an online diet program will come with an interactive meal program. This is where you can enter in the foods that you like and the meal planner will create you a menu for the next few weeks. These are very helpful and will be able to save you a lot of time, which you would have spent on the caloric counting value of each meal.

There is also a degree of flexibility that is available online, which your local program will not be able to provide you. Instead of you having to attend a meeting once a week you will be able to track your weight loss on your own time schedule.

You are the only one who knows which program will work best for you. You need to decide what your needs are and do careful research on each aspect. Choosing a proper weight loss program, that works for you; will help you achieve your goals.

Before and After Success Stories

What happens after you diet? Weight loss before and after stories are common. When you lose a significant amount of weight, your life can change in many pleasant ways. Here is some weight loss before and after stories.

Margie had gained 30 pounds after her second pregnancy. She was sluggish – and not just because she had to keep up with a baby and a toddler. She felt that her weight was keeping her from being the mother she wanted to be.

Margie went to a dietitian to help her change her food choices. One of the things Susan, her dietitian, suggested was to eat a variety of whole foods that were low in fat and high in fiber. Margie had been making a variety of quick meals and picking up fast food because of her duties as a mom. She decided that it was important to start cooking wholesome meals for her husband and herself. She quickly started losing one to two pounds a week. Within 4 months, she was back to her pre-pregnancy weight. What a great weight loss before & after story.

Another factor that was important in her weight loss she wanted to create a family of healthy eaters. She didn't want her kids to think that food came from McDonalds. Fast food should be an occasional treat not a mainstay of their diets.

Margie's weight loss before & after story is an inspiration to all new moms struggling to lose the baby weight.

Rob was a teacher at an exclusive public school who has his own weight loss before & after story. One of the perks of teaching at the school was that it provided a catered lunch each day. In addition, fellow teachers often brought specialty foods to share at lunchtime.

The camaraderie in the lunchroom was one of the strengths of the school program. But it was killing Rob's waistline. He decided that he would bring a low calorie sack lunch and begin walking during 20 minutes of his lunch break. He worried that skipping the lunchroom would mean he would distance himself from his fellow teachers. But, when they saw that he was losing a significant amount of weight on his program, many of the other teachers joined in. Soon, there was a teacher's walking club at lunch time. A "club" based around an unhealthy eating pattern was replaced by one based on a healthy one.

What a wonderful weight loss before & after story!

Kerry was a busy mom with a 50+ hour a week job. When she wasn't working, she wanted to spend time with her two boys, Gregg who was 9 and Vince who was 11. She felt guilty about going to the gym because that was an hour and a half she could have been spending with her kids.

But, as she crept up near 200 pounds, she knew something had to change. One thing she did was get up a half hour earlier in the morning to take a walk. Then, when she got home in the evenings, she made a point of playing 20 minutes of basketball with the boys every day. Her new physical activity combined with a low fat, lower calorie diet, led to her losing 55 pounds over the course of a year.

Being able to increase the time she spent with her kids as well as losing the weight was a win-win for Kerry. That's a truly great weight loss before & after story.

Do you have your own weight loss before & after story? Be sure to share it with others as it can encourage them to lose weight as well.

Key Elements Of Long Term Weight Loss

You are probably trying to lose weight, but you are trying to figure out how to lose your weight, for a longer time period than just a few months. There are a lot of programs out there that provide you with many tips and ideas but most of these make false promises and do not deliver. Still others may tell you that you will lose weight for long terms but you find yourself just after a few months slowly climbing up the weight scale. However there are a few key elements that you can look at that will help you achieve your long term weight loss goals.

1. Health

* You will probably agree with someone who says that your health is one of your most valuable assets. If you are feeling sad or unhappy you will probably want to take the time to build and maintain your health before you begin your weight loss program. If you have good health it will be the starting point for many great weight loss results.

75

2. Competing with yourself

* Are you one of those that compare themselves to someone else? This is not a good concept for you to follow instead you need to compete with yourself and not anyone else. Only you can select the results that you are looking for. You must remember you are the one that will be setting your weight loss goals not someone else. You will also be the one that is motivating yourself.

3. Lifestyle

* Improvement in your weight or even fitness is all about you creating something great or giving something up. In order for you to reach your weight loss goals and stay there you are going to have to make some important lifestyle changes. With positive reinforcement your weight loss will become a commitment that you will make to yourself. Once you make it a habit you will see yourself losing the weight and keeping it off.

4. Start Now

* You need to start your weight loss program right away. You need to develop the mind frame it's never too late to start motto and you will be well on your way to reaching your goals. Setting

goals and meeting them is one of the best rewards that you will be able to do for yourself.

5. Grateful

* Take time to be grateful for the things you have and the weight you have already lost. Taking time to feel grateful will make you feel better about yourself which is important when you are trying to lose weight.

As you can see most of these elements deal with a lifestyle change. You need to change certain aspects of your life to achieve your long term weight loss goals. If you are willing to do this then you will be successful in your goals.

Looking and Feeling Good Summary

When it comes to body weight, many women face a struggle; an uphill battle. Faced with images of optimal health and physical perfection in advertisements, in films and on television, it's easy to slip into a rut of inadequacy. It's very easy to forget that those images are heavily edited and Photoshopped.

But take a few moments to sit and watch the world; look at those who walk past. You won't see flawless perfection. You'll see real humans, complete with flaws and flab.

Some look at the thin, beautiful models in advertisements and find the inspiration and drive to reinvent and self-transform. These people are inspired by people whom they admire and wish to emulate.

Others look at people who are overweight and less-than-perfect and they too find the drive to self-improve and they're inspired by those who represent that which they do not want to become.

But in order to be successful in looking and feeling your very best, it's important to find a motivation and inspiration that's rooted within yourself. Don't aspire to be like someone else. And don't aspire to be the antithesis of that which you loathe. Aspire to be the best version of you! It's these people who are the most successful when it comes to losing weight, looking great and truly appreciating the reflection in the mirror.

That's the first and most fundamental key when it comes to looking and feeling good! Don't aspire to be someone else; aspire to be the best version of yourself! And realize that nobody is perfect; everyone has flaws. Don't let those flaws prevent you from loving yourself. Life is a journey. It's important to enjoy the journey and find happiness along the way; don't postpone happiness until you arrive at the destination.

Quite simply, looking and feeling good is not about impressing others. In fact, those who try to lose weight or change for others rarely sustain that change in the long term. "Looking and feeling good" is about creating a version of yourself that appeal to you; it's about what makes you happy. To truly look good, you must go beyond the physical and that which is skin deep; it's about self-love, happiness and confidence!

The Dynamics of Obesity and Weight Loss

According to the U.S. Center for Disease Control (CDC), you're not alone if you're struggling with your weight. More than one-third of American adults are obese. More than 35 percent of Americans are considered obese and as a result, more than a third of Americans are more susceptible to type two diabetes, high blood pressure, heart disease, joint pain and joint degradation, stroke and even some forms of cancer. So losing weight, exercising and getting healthy go far beyond aesthetics; for many, it's a matter of long term survival!

In the simplest terms, being overweight or obese arises as a result of an energy imbalance. Your body requires energy --- in the form of calories --- to survive and thrive! Calories are the fuel that drives the human body.

But an energy imbalance arises when the amount of calories consumed exceeds the amount of calories that are expended. So in order to remedy this, you must exercise and eat a healthy diet that's lower in calories or fat. To lose weight, you must expend more calories than you consume on a daily basis.

But many make the mistake of believing that you can starve yourself thin by severely limiting food intake. In reality, this has an adverse impact on your health. What's more, it's extremely difficult to lose weight using this approach; long term weight loss utilizing this method is even more challenging --- and this refers only to the physical aspects of starvation. This says nothing about the mental and spiritual experience of self-imposed starvation, which is extremely taxing and very unhealthy.

You see, the body is dynamic. If you severely limit the amount of food that you consume, your body's metabolism shifts to accommodate the apparent period of starvation. Once your body shifts into starvation mode, your metabolism slows to a crawl. Your body alters the way it functions in order to conserve energy. Your energy levels drop to an all-time low. You're always tired and sleepy. Even your digestive system slows so it can absorb more calories and nutrients from each meal. Simply getting through the day is difficult; exercising seems impossible!

Quite simply, starving yourself isn't the solution. The moment you resume eating --- and you must resume eating or you simply won't survive --- you'll be faced with the challenge of speeding up your super slow metabolism. Your metabolism can shift into starvation mode fairly quickly, but shifting from starvation mode to normal mode is a much slower process. It's a process that takes time and as a result, many gain weight even more rapidly than they did previously! Plus, you've failed to make any major changes in terms of diet and lifestyle, which means you'll continue to gain weight as you did before you went on your 'diet.'

What are the net results of the starvation diet? You <u>feel</u> terrible. Mentally, you're *constantly* craving food. Spiritually, you're exhausted. And you're apt to look terrible too! Sure, you may be a bit lighter, but your skin will appear sallow, your energy will be sapped; even your hair will take on a thin, dead appearance. And your metabolism is slower than ever, so the moment you resume eating, you're faced with even more rapid weight gain!

So this leads us to the first rule when it comes to looking and feeling good.

Looking and Feeling Good Tip 01: To gain energy and reduce cravings you have to EAT

That's right! You must eat in order to lose weight, reduce cravings and gain energy!

Losing weight isn't about suffering and going without for a short period of time in order to lose weight; that's simply not sustainable, nor is it healthy.

The key to long term weight loss and a healthy physique is a healthy diet!

One of the first keys to gaining energy and reducing cravings is to eat often. Instead of eating two or three large meals each day, eat smaller, more frequent meals. Eating five to six meals per day speeds your metabolism, which promotes more rapid calorie consumption by your body and this is what leads to weight loss!

More frequent meals also provide you with more energy because your blood sugar levels will be more constant; there will be fewer peaks and valleys. Well-moderated blood sugar is key to looking and feeling great! What's more, maintaining more stable, healthier blood sugar levels can serve to reverse the effects of obesity as it relates to "type two diabetes"! So you won't just feel healthier, you'll actually be healthier!

Eating more frequent meals will knock out those cravings too! Cravings are rooted in hunger and nutritional deficiencies. And while cravings can take on an intense psychological role in the weight loss process, it's much easier to resist those cravings when you're feeling full. More frequent meals will also serve to prevent binge eating, since you'll no longer experience the extreme hunger that drives binge eating.

While it is important to eat often, it's also important to eat a balanced diet too! Nutritional deficiencies are a powerful element in the weight loss equation. Cravings are a natural biological mechanism for driving you to eat foods that will serve to correct those deficiencies. That's why many women experience intense cravings when they opt for exclusion diets, which are diets that exclude one or more major food type (often, carbohydrate-rich foods.)

Quite simply, when you eat a balanced diet, those nutritional deficiencies should be corrected and as a result, your cravings will diminish. Many women take a multivitamin too, as this provides added coverage to ensure your body is receiving the nutrients it needs to thrive!

Once your body receives the nutrients and calories it needs to perform at an optimal level, you'll feel the difference. You'll enjoy increased energy levels (perfect for taking on a healthy exercise routine!), reduced cravings, enhanced concentration and more emotional stability. Yes, poor nutrition can impact your mind, your cognition and your emotions quite dramatically!

In sum, eating a balanced variety of foods in lots of small, frequent meals throughout the day is a first step toward looking good and feeling great!

Looking And Feeling Good Tip 02:
Find --- Then Eat --- The Good Carbs!

Carbohydrates or 'carbs' are often excluded, as many women are under the (false) impression that carbs promote weight gain and/or hinder weight loss efforts. This isn't true. And excluding all carbs from your diet can result not only in nutritional deficiencies; it can also result in intense cravings, which often have a dramatic impact on your mood and overall sense of wellness! Nobody wants to feel deprived! And these feelings of deprivation can leave us feeling ravenous for carbs!

When you're overcome by cravings and left feeling not-so-fabulous, it's virtually impossible to *look* good when you *feel* terrible!

So, the key to a healthy diet that promotes weight loss: Don't exclude all carbs! Exclude the unhealthy carbs; eat the healthy carbs. A simple task, if you understand which carbs are 'good' and which carbs are 'bad.'

Carbs are found in grains, fruits and vegetables. Quite simply, foods with 'good carbs' also have lots of fiber present, while 'bad carbs' have the fiber stripped away as a result of processing or refining.

'Bad carbs' are found in foods like white bread, white rice, potato chips and fries.

'Good carbs' are found in foods like whole grain bread, brown rice, beans, carrots and other fruits and veggies.

Generally, look for carbs that have not undergone lots of processing or refinement. If they've been processed, they'll often fall into the category of 'bad carbs.'

And, as always, moderation is key! Women should get 45 to 65 percent of their calories from carbs (along with 20 to 35 percent from fat and 10 to 35 percent from protein. Generally, when you're looking to lose weight, you should eat less fat and more protein, which helps you to develop muscle during your exercise and fitness routine!)

Carbs make you feel satisfied, which is very important with your meals! If you're not feeling satisfied, then you're apt to suffer from cravings and other adverse psychological effects.

These are the keys to looking and feeling good! It all comes from within! Eating a healthy diet, combined with a great exercise and fitness routine, will give you the energy you need to power through your day, while losing weight and maintaining a great attitude!

Looking And Feeling Good Tip 03: Thoughts on Exercise- Just do it!

Now we get to the heart of what it takes to change you from the inside out. Yes, it the dreaded word "Exercise". This is where we must exert just a little effort to achieve small gains that with continued effort may turn into much larger gains, which will move us from where we reside to creating the inner and outer body we desire.

I will admit that it sounds good, but we both know that anything worth having requires dedication, force of will and a never give up attitude. We all have what it takes to accomplish anything we want. So what happens to us when we jump in that first day, week or month? If we don't see or feel that we are changing or exercise is helping we quit.

Your body will do anything you tell it to. But your mind, your friends, even your family may plant ideas in your mind that you can't or won't stay to path. All of the excuses will rush into your mind and there you are on the edges of becoming the biggest loser. When you start to think like that you will feel like saying "What the use", "Who am I fooling". You might say to yourself "I'm only human".

Dose any of this ring any bells. If you are honest with yourself, you know of what I speak. You are not alone. There are millions who fall into that state of mind. Why do you think we are a culture of "quick fits" and "I want it now". We have been program and lead to that fountain and we have all taken a sip. Very few of us stay the path and really understand what it takes to sustain looking and feeling good. Some of us have no choice; we must always dedicate ourselves to looking good and therefore feeling good. Why is that you said. The answer is because they have to do everything they can each and every day to keep themselves on the path or they will not have a job or career.

I am not talking about athletes, actors and actresses, but people in the corporate world too. They all have the desire to continually fight the mental pings of giving into that small voice that says, "Why continue to torture yourself", "Who cares?

I am not talking about setting goals or New Year Resolutions. I am talking about a lifestyle. One where you have the information you need to make a change in your life. Do the things that make you happy, health and looking good and feeling good. Be the leader, manager, director and the president of you. If you are able to take control and you can, just decide to be on the path to discovering "How to look and feel good".

Looking And Feeling Good Tip 04: Take the Journey

And remember, whatever your weight, love yourself! Be confident! Nobody is perfect. Embrace your flaws, and find hope and motivation as you work to improve! This will enable you to enjoy the journey; even if you never make it to your intended destination.

One LastThank You Again!

I really appreciate your support with this book and I really hope that you have gone through it; it will help you achieve the success you desire.

Just a reminder if you have time

Now that you have gone through the book, if you get a free second could you post your honest review on Amazon.com? Reviews from honest people like you help me further develop future books so that I can help more people just like you.

Looking And Feeling Good Series

If you liked this book then you will love the rest of the books in the above series.

Coming Soon:

Exercise Tips For Weight Loss

Examine many aspect of weight loss through the various types and kinds of exercises. This book will provide information that you can apply in your effort to determine which form and type will aid your journey to achieve the results you desire.

Diet Programs For Weight Loss

There are vast array of Diet Programs. We are bombarded each and every day in various medias aimed at attracting and holding your attention. The question is "Which one is best for you? You are provided information that may help you to make an informed decision.

94

www.ingramcontent.com/pod-product-compliance
Lightning Source LLC
Chambersburg PA
CBHW052055270326
41931CB00012B/2771